UNCOMFORTABLE
PEACE

Stepping Outside My Comfort Zone to Naturally Beat Type 2 Diabetes

Vernon P. Davis Jr.

Contributing Editor: Carol Curley-Davis

Foreword by Kemia Carter, MS, RDN, LDN

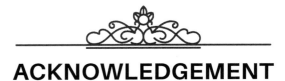

ACKNOWLEDGEMENT

I want to thank God for being by my side through this scary period of my life and seeing me through it. I thank God for making the fruits, veggies and herbs that healed and saved my body.

To my Wife of whom has supported me even before I was diagnosed, I thank you and love you. To my Son, my motivation to get better, thank you, Daddy loves you. To my Mom, Dad, Brother and Sister who kept me encouraged each day and supported me, I love you. To my in-laws for keeping me encouraged, I love you. To my cousin Lawrence who made changes with me so I wasn't alone, thank you and I love you. To all my family and friends that talked with me, prayed with/for me and cheered me on, thank you. To my friends in the medical field, Ari and Rine, thank you both for supporting me and assisting me along this journey.

To Tony Lee and Brione Reid, thank you both for your knowledge and field of study. You two have aided me in a tough battle. I wouldn't be on the other side of this illness without you guys and your expertise.

Lastly, I want to thank Dr. Sebi, may your teachings continue to aid in the healing of others.

DEDICATION

This book is dedicated to anyone challenged with type 2 diabetes or prediabetes and desires to improve his or her health naturally.

FOREWORD

Greetings! My name is Kemia Carter, MS, RDN, LDN. I am a registered dietitian nutritionist and licensed dietitian nutritionist. I received both my Bachelor's and Master's degrees in Nutritional Science and Dietetics respectfully from Texas Tech University. My passion for math, chemistry and food has expedited my career in nutrition since a young girl in elementary.

Upon graduating high school, my paternal grandfather became ill due to his diagnosis of type 2 diabetes. With resistance to implementing healthy lifestyle changes and improving his eating habits, he became my guardian angel. From that day on, I made a promise to myself that I would make an impact on the world with God-given gifts to assist and educate others on beneficial nutrition interventions and using food as medicine. Nutrition interests include weight management, chronic disease prevention, renal, pediatric, oncology, and sports nutrition.

It has been my pleasure to know Vernon Davis for the past five years. I was introduced to Vernon through a relationship with one of his family members and the rest is history! In short, I would describe my first impression of Vernon as confident, calm and humble. His honesty and transparency are admirable as well as his continuous journey to optimal health.

Type 2 diabetes, although a chronic illness, is self-inflicted for most people. Poor nutrition choices, lack of sufficient hydration and inadequate discipline caused Vernon to be counted among the roughly 30 million Americans diagnosed with this disease. With self-education, accountability partners and consistent conversations with the man in the mirror, Vernon not only reversed type 2 diabetes naturally but lives to spread his testimony.

Vernon's motivation for forging a path to type 2 diabetes reversal and reaching optimal health include: enhancing nutrition knowledge through extensive research. Secondly, focusing on the prioritization of personal health goals one decision at a time. Third, taking necessary actions to exercise healthy behaviors day-to-day. Lastly, avoiding side effects of a primarily pharmaceutical approach.

I am honored to enlighten you all on a miraculous transformation of mind, body and spirit. It is in great confidence that I illuminate the immediate changes Mr. Davis made upon learning the current status of his health. You can expect to gain motivation and clear direction on where to begin your research after understanding the journey that Vernon has chosen to a healthier life.
Yours truly,

Kemia Carter, MS, RDN, LDN

Table of Contents

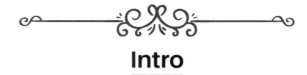

Intro

"Nephew, sometimes we go through things in life not for ourselves but so that once we overcome, we can then aid others in getting through the same thing." Those were the words of my Uncle Keith back in 2012 when I developed an abscess on my face. I remember being in the clinic getting it drained thinking, "why me, Lord?" I had just graduated from Grambling State University and relocated to Virginia for the next chapter of my life. Who knew his words would ring consistently in my head a decade later as I worked to overcome type 2 diabetes?

This book is documentation of my journey to fighting one of the scariest, yet quite familiar, illnesses in our country. What I have to share is not medical advice, I'm no doctor. In fact, for anything you find informative in this book, I would advise consulting a physician prior to implementing. What I have to share is my story, the actions I took to improve my own health and not rely solely on the opinion of others.

My prayer over this writing is that it can be a catalyst for other diabetics in working toward reversing this illness in their bodies.

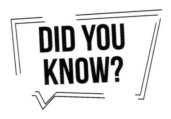

- "34.2 Million Americans have diabetes"
- Over 90% are Type 2
- Only 25% are aware

Source:

https://www.cdc.gov/chronicdisease/resources/publications/factsheets/
diabetes-prediabetes.htm

My view on my own health

As a child I ate a lot, I played a lot and I slept a lot. I enjoyed cheese and barbeque flavored chips; my father worked for a global manufacturer of chips and assorted snacks. I loved my great grandmothers baked macaroni and cheese. My grandmothers and aunts all knew their way around the kitchen, and I knew how to clean a plate. As I got older, more independent and gained more access to food, I indulged. I would always hear about how too much of this or that can harm your body long term, but I didn't think that applied to me. Surely God wouldn't let me get sick or develop an illness from the foods I loved. I mean, I always prayed for God to "please bless this meal, remove any impurities, make it a blessing and nourishment to my body…" Little did I know, in a way I was mocking God and had yet to realize it.

Basketball and weights were my exercises of choice. I wasn't stellar at either, but I knew basics and enjoyed contributing to a group in play or competition. I always figured if I stayed active, along with my prayers over my food, that I couldn't get any short term nor long term illness from what I ate; sweaty activity and faith just had to be the recipe for staying off the "sick and shut-in list". When I reflect on how many sports figures and models graced our television screen on commercials for popular fast food restaurants, I just knew that if they looked that great of shape and ate that stuff, surely if I maintained a simple sweating regimen then I could eat whatever I wanted to and keep a clean bill of health.

Questions:

1. How do you view your health?

2. What does it mean to be healthy, to you?

My Eating habits

"Now be sure to use this food up and pack your lunch for tomorrow. Don't forget an apple or plum to go with it. Don't take more than one bag of chips". These are the words of my parents to my siblings and me week after week growing up. They had no understanding that the cool kids purchased lunch at school: nachos, pizza, chicken tenders, pasta, rolls, cake, ice cream cups, and a soda or juice: these were the menu items every day in middle school and high school. After a long 4-5 hours of learning, something tasty was needed to refuel and finish out the day.

As a teenager, I ate many times through the day: breakfast at home, breakfast at school, a quick snack from the school store and a hand full of chips from a friend. This was all before 1st period. Food was always on my mind. If there was an event I asked if refreshments were provided. If my family and I were going somewhere I asked if we were stopping to get something to eat while being out. I learned through my own experiences that if nothing else could soothe me or offset any negatives emotions, food could. Without knowing at the time, I was living to eat.

Things took a turn for the worst after high school graduation: college cafeterias! When I arrived to campus, I learned very quickly that my three meals a day in the Café were all buffet style. There were different cultural meals offered daily but the pizza bar, fried chicken and dessert station were consistent for lunch and dinner. I enjoyed pancakes, sausage, bacon, with grits and eggs every morning. Whether the crew intended on dining at 7am or not, I was not missing out!

I wasn't aware of food delivery apps back in undergrad, but I was fortunate to know others with vehicles. "Hey Carl, want to drive into town to grab a burger, I'm buying". This was a regular sentence I uttered to friends and classmates until I had my own vehicle to get around it. I didn't hesitate to offer food because I learned that five dollars for gas was not enticing to vehicle owners for a 30–45-minute trip at 9pm in the evening.

After college on through 2020, I maintained a pretty physical relationship with food, so much that it resembled an affair. If I had a problem with someone or something, I would go to the kitchen or corner store or a nearby restaurant to get something to eat to subside my frustrations, instead of dealing with the issue and searching for resolution. Snowstorms and tornadoes were scary, but I hadn't much experience with those in my life. When I began experiencing them in Virginia, I always ran to either a grocery store to stock up on junk food or bought a big meal I could eat on for a few days. Now I'm not saying this is horrible to do, I believe there is wisdom in being prepared for a storm. What I'm saying is, food was the one thing I would run to in a moment of fear and uncertainty because I knew it could soothe and comfort me.

Questions:

1. What are your eating habits?

2. What are reasons besides hunger that you choose to eat?

3. How do you determine that you are hungry?

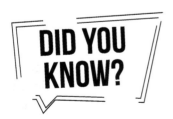

"Diabetes can also lead to amputation of a limb, loss of vision and kidney failure."

Source:

https://www.cdc.gov/chronicdisease/resources/publications/factsheets/diabetes-prediabetes.htm

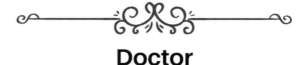

Doctor

In 2019 I married the love of my life! After our honeymoon she began noticing things about me that I never gave much thought to. I had always claimed to be a light sleeper and to a degree that is true. I would get up constantly through the night to potty and snack. My wife noticed my habits and mentioned them. I didn't think much of it, but she did. When we were dating we would share meals intentionally: my wife didn't eat much as in it didn't take much for her to get satisfied and I was working out with a trainer to lose weight, so it was in my best interest to not consume an entire meal but to split it with my wife. What my wife learned about me after we got married was that I would stop at fast food restaurants after escorting her home from our dates.

My wife also noticed that I slowly began missing her calls on my off days. I would be home asleep and would not hear my ringer which was uncommon for me. "You probably should go see a doctor," she'd say. Now this isn't the first time she has recommended that I go get a check-up, but it is the first time she had mentioned it to which I had no excuse not to go. See, throughout our relationship I held several jobs. I worked at a hotel that I loved. On my off days I was on call. I had no health insurance, so a medical visit had to be an absolute emergency for me. I accepted a management/training role with a fast-food company that allotted me two consecutive days off a week; but the mental stress made it difficult for me to do errands on those days, let alone make an appointment and actually go. So, I never did. Not even with them offering health insurance. Mind you, I maintained a consistent workout regime with a trainer, so I had that excuse going for me as well. Shortly after leaving that training position, I accepted a management position with another company that required 75% travel. I felt like I couldn't make a doctor's appointment since I was not sure if I would be in town for it even though their health insurance was better than my previous employer. Moreover, my superior always did his very best to accommodate my schedule, but again, I made the excuse. In February 2019 I became unemployed and had no intention of spending what little money I had considering our wedding was 4 months away.

Prior to our union, I accepted the role with my current employer whom offered the best benefit package I've had since aging off my dad's insurance. I had set days off that I could plan around. I had no excuse now for refusing to see a doctor at my wife's request. I remember going in September of 2019 and getting a routine physical. I was 285lbs with an elevated blood pressure. Dr. R recommended I follow the *dash diet*, a plan I had never heard of. He wanted to setup another appointment to get some blood work that would test my A1c level. We scheduled for December. I don't remember what happened, but I cancelled the appointment and did not make it in to get blood work done until April of 2020.

Questions:

1. When is you next Dr appointment?

2. What were the results of your last Dr. appointment?

3. What excuse, if any, have you made to not go see a Dr?

Pandemic

It was a typical day at the office. I strolled into work to get a good spot in the refrigerator for my spaghetti. I filled my container with ice and water. I made my multiday purchase of sour worms from the convenience store in the break area, and I logged into my computer ready to tackle the day. Slowly I noticed my colleagues packing their desk and taking all they could carry out the door. I then received a call from my immediate superior. "The pandemic numbers are increasing rapidly, we have decided it is in your best interest to have you service our clients from home. Take all you need, here is all the company technology you need and stay safe". The pandemic afforded many Americans with the opportunity to work from home. The challenge for me was being home alone with a kitchen full of food. Going into the office I carried a lunch bag and limited myself to only purchasing candy to snack on. Working from home allowed me instant access to 3-5 servings of leftovers, a 64-ounce carton of juice, cookies and candy and anything else we purchased on our biweekly grocery store visit. As the weeks progressed as I'm working from home, little did I know I was eating myself into an early grave. After a few weeks working from home, I went back to Dr. R to get my blood drawn for analysis. The follow up appointment scheduled for the next week was cancelled at his request due to the rising cases of Covid. This went on for 3 months, from April to July. I didn't care too much; I did not want to know the results. "Can't have a problem if you don't know about the problem."

Ironically during those 3 months, I would urinate consistently during the day and break my sleep multiple times throughout the night to go as well. I was always thirsty so I drank at least a gallon of soda and juice along with a gallon of water.....to balance everything out ☺. I also experienced consistent numbness and tingling in my fingers and toes, but I always thought it was due to keeping the home cold.

Questions:

1. Since the pandemic, how have your eating habits changed?

2. Have you noticed anything "off" about your body?

3. If you have, have you gone to see a medical professional?

Offutt Wedding

In July of 2020, my best friend and her husband were due to say "I do" in front of a crowd of friends and family. I was honored to participate as a groomsman. Prior to their wedding, Dr. R had called to confirm the follow up appointment that had been set for me to finally come see him about my blood work results. The date of the appointment was shortly after the wedding. I promised my wife I would go. Before the appointment I noticed a bit more of how out of whack my body really was. The Offutt wedding was in the state of Michigan, about an 11-hour drive from us. We broke the drive up into 2 stints. We departed on a Friday evening and rested in Pennsylvania. I remember stopping every hour to urinate and to get a $1.00 32-ounce drink from a national fast-food restaurant. The next morning we continued on, at this point of the trip I noticed just how weak my bladder was. Several times I pulled over on the side of the highway to relieve myself because I felt as though I could not make it to the next gas station. My wife was worried but I assured her I had just drunk too much juice…all the while heading to get another beverage as we continued on our journey.

Once in Dearborn, I began to think through my issues and concluded that I had to do whatever I could to ensure that I didn't ruin my friend's wedding by having the need to step away and urinate. Once we checked into our hotel at 3pm, I decided that I was not going to drink anything past 7pm so that I had no reason to need to urinate during the wedding ceremony the next day. That plan had holes I didn't see coming. Saturday evening, the groom and his groomsman all went out for a night on the town to see the area. I must say, it was beautiful. But I could not enjoy it fully due to my bladder. Sadly, I had to separate from the group and rush to a restroom, any restroom before I wet my pants. Covid protocol slowed me down, with taking temperatures, getting a visitors pass and then waiting for a stall to open. I held it just long enough to not embarrass myself any more than what I had. After the sigh of relief, it was time for me to head back to the hotel. I had to be in range of a toilet so I could get everything out before the wedding.

The wedding day was fun, the morning was eventful, and my bladder kept requiring disposal. I learned that not only were we riding on a party bus as a wedding party, but also that the outdoor location had no restroom. I was in shock. Why? Because although I hadn't drunk anything since 7pm the night before, I was still rushing to unzip and relieve. Prior to meeting the wedding party at the bus pickup location, I drove to a parking lot nearby, A PARKING LOT, and urinated behind a dumpster…. a dumpster. I unfastened my groomsman outfit just to release. At this point I began to really worry about my body. Horrible timing since I was in a wedding that was about to begin.

The wedding was beautiful, I mean flawless! Once it ended the wedding party was loading up to cruise the city before photos. Guess what I got to do? Yes, you guessed it. I hopped into my vehicle and raced to find a place to urinate. It was sad, very sad. After photos, my wife and I hit the road back to Pennsylvania with a crazy amount of urination stops along the way. It was like I had to urinate just as much without drinking anything as I did when I was loaded on fluids. My wife, in her brilliance, triple checked that I was going to the doctor for my upcoming appointment.

Questions:

1. Again I ask: are there any crazy changes to your body that you have noticed?

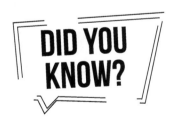

Globally, Asians make up 60% of the diabetes population.

Source:

https://asiandiabetesprevention.org/what-is-diabetes/why-are-asians-higher-risk

Diagnosed

Well, I was 24 hours away from not only getting an update but also to asking questions about what is going on with me. I was not looking forward to seeing Dr. R because I knew I was going to get some kind of bad news. Well, the pandemic caused Dr. R to reschedule my appointment yet again. In a way I felt a sense of relief in not finding out any bad news that week. Well as you might imagine, my wife was not going for that. "Ok, so Dr. R won't see you tomorrow, but you are going somewhere to get checked out. The excessive urinating, the constant tingling in your fingers, toes and legs, the dry mouth and constantly being thirsty not to mention always being tired and sluggish. Oh, you are going somewhere tomorrow to get checked out, let me know when you figure it out."

Well the Queen had spoken and I had to find somewhere to go to at least express my concerns about the symptoms I had been displaying the last few months, not to mention the last 7 days. I settled on going to a local clinic the following morning when they opened. My wife was well pleased.

The next morning after my wife left for work, I left to go to the clinic. Knowing that I would most likely get some bad news and even be put on some restrictions, I prepared myself. I stopped by a local gas station to get a slush and four of their $1.00 fountain drinks, two were sodas and the other two were fruit punch. I didn't get them to drink before I went in the clinic; I couldn't sabotage any numbers like that. I got them so that after hearing whatever bad news they gave me whether a medical assumption or concrete fact, I needed to have something in my car ready to consume to soothe me. This is how bad it was for me in finding comfort in food and sugary drinks.

Upon my arrival to the clinic, I prayed for the best outcome and went in with my head held high; convincing myself that there was not anything too bad with me. After sharing with the doctor my symptoms and getting a physical and blood/urine work, the doctor casually expressed "well you are urinating frequently with the feeling of not being able to hold it because you are type 2 diabetic". With a shaking voice I asked, "excuse me, I am what." "You are a type 2 diabetic, your A1c is off the charts, over 15.5 which is the highest we can measure, and your blood sugar level is 476 which is scary." "How scary," I asked. "You should be in an emergency room right now, it's a shock you were able to drive here. Have you experienced being lightheaded or blurred vision?" I paused before responding; I knew the answer but I had yet to share those things with my wife. I figured now was not the time to hold back, I was just told I had "the sugars" so I replied, "yes I have had trouble focusing at times. My left eye was the worse, not being able to make out simple shapes and figures at random times. I would get lightheaded periodically throughout the day as well."

The doctor was very calm in his speech; I guess they give this diagnosis on a regular basis. He told me I needed to lay off anything with added sugar, gave me a prescription for a certain diabetes medication and advised me to get a glucose meter and test strips. I googled the medication the doctor prescribed and became fearful of the side effects. I took the prescription paperwork and held it together as I departed the building.

Data: Weight, 275lbs. Glucose reading, 476. A1C **Greater Than** 15.5

Questions:

1. Have you been diagnosed with diabetes?

2. Do you know your A1C level and Blood sugar level?

3. How did you feel when you found out?

4. If you have not been diagnosed but suspect that you could be diabetic, what symptoms have you been displaying and what is holding you back from finding out?

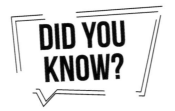

In 2017, diabetes was mentioned as a cause of death in a total of 270,702 death certificates

Source:

https://www.diabetes.org/resources/statistics/statistics-about-diabetes

Godly Herbs.com

As I walked out the door, the tears began flowing. I called my mom and could hardly get it out, my voice was cracking bad. I told her everything and she told me she loved me and that she would do whatever she could to help me. She was over 1,000 miles away.

After speaking with her I called my wife who cried with me, she was hurt because I was hurting and she doesn't want anything to happen to me, we don't want to lose each other. As she prayed for me, I took one sip from one of my five drinks and threw them all away. I had to make a change and that was the start. I had no clue what to do moving forward. I told my wife I loved her and I remembered the physical transformation that one of my friends had in a 3-4 month span.

After hanging up with my wife I called my friend Brione, of Godlyherbs.com. I explained to him what I had just found out and he smile and offered great encouragement, reassuring me that there was a way to get my health back on track naturally. He began to explain to me what he had learned and implemented from his own research of herbalists over the years, eating alkaline foods and avoiding acidic foods. He also made mention of consuming natural herbs and sea vegetables to help heal the body. I had never heard of natural herbs and sea vegetables but I was desperate and so I was open to trying anything natural. I refused to use the prescribed diabetes medication and so I never did…EVER.

Later in this book I will go into detail of the natural herbs and sea vegetables.

Now eating was just a piece of the pie. I also needed to get serious about sweating, shedding a few pounds. There was one person I could call, one person that I trusted to get me where I needed to be.

Questions:

1. If you take prescription medication, what side effects are you experiencing?

2. Is prescription medication helping you reach your goals?

3. Have you considered adding natural herbs, plants and sea vegetables to your regime?

AEL Fitness

Once Brione and I hung up, I gave a call to Mr. Tony Lee of Aneducatorlifestyle.com. Mr. Lee had been my trainer for years, and while I had seen great success in getting stronger, I hadn't loss much weight due to my eating habits.

Still in the parking lot of the clinic, I spoke with Mr. Lee and explained to him the news. He too was calm and encouraging, letting me know that he would put together a regimen for me to help combat this illness and that due to the pandemic we would have to work out virtually. He reassured me that he knew what he had to offer would benefit me and that all I had to do was follow his guidance and recommendations. I was not a fan of working out virtually but I was desperate, so I agreed. I let him know that I would be ready to start in 2 weeks, I needed to detox my body first. He explained that although this would not be easy, the hardest part had been done- committing to the process.

After beginning my detox, I changed my mind. Instead of waiting 2 weeks to get started, we began a week later and it was one of the better decisions as it relates to small victories and overcoming my own mind, which can get in our way of change and success.

Questions:

1. If you are diabetic or suspect that you might be, what are your views on exercising to help combat the illness?

2. What routine do you use if you are working out?

3. Do you workout alone? Why or why not?

4. Have you purchased Tony Lees book, *"Prioritizing You: Combatting The Common Excuses"*? It is available on Amazon.

Research mode

After hanging up with Mr. Lee and Brione, I went straight to my local pharmacy to get the diabetes medication prescription filled. I was in tears just standing in line trying to wrap my mind around my reality. The pharmacy tech took my prescription, looked at me and concluded I was just diagnosed. He was very encouraging, saying that his mom had to take it and got her numbers down. She was able to get off the medication after a few years. Hearing that made me cry more. I accepted the pills then headed home.

Now home, still in tears, I'm met by my loving wife who took the rest of the day off to be with me and comfort me. There came a point where I had to get up and stop feeling sorry for myself. I had work to do. As much as I believed what the doctor told me about my diagnosis, I was not as accepting of the steps to get better.

After calming down, I used the search engine on my cell phone to see what the side effects of this medication was: diarrhea, vomiting, nausea, chest discomfort, headaches, dehydration, shortness of breath, nerve damage, and lactic acidosis which could lead to a rapid heart rate, and even death. After praying to God about what I read and the change that I desired. I made a personal decision to take ownership of my situation and opted not to take the prescribed medication or sign up for the education class that was offered by the local hospital. In fact, I threw the medication away immediately. I concluded that the steps I take would have to be based on my own conviction and I could not do that without researching natural alternatives.

After researching diabetes and the national statistics, I began to investigate the herbalist that Brione made mention of, Dr. Sebi. If you haven't heard of him, I would implore you to look him up. Dr. Sebi made a bold statement in a video I saw on the Internet: "The Mucus membrane being compromised is the cause of all diseases. Eliminating the excess mucus will eliminate the disease in the part of the body that has the compromised mucus membrane." According to Dr. Sebi, my pancreatic ducts had excess mucus causing me to be insulin resistant. This also had a negative effect on my kidneys and liver, so getting this illness out my body was going to benefit multiple organs, not just one. Dr. Sebi taught me that clearing my body at an intracellular level was priority and recommended that I consume natural herbs and sea moss to make myself well. In addition to that, he recommended eating alkaline foods. Brione and I spoke more concerning these things and he helped me begin looking into the natural items that could be beneficial for me.

I learned a bit more about the body and pH level during my research. I learned that the body functions best when its pH level is balanced. In order to maintain a balanced pH I had to eat foods that promoted alkalinity in the body. Alkalinity combats acidification and acidification for me was the fostering of an acidic environment in my body. Diseases thrive in an acidic environment but cannot survive in an alkaline environment. With this, the information Brione shared, plus what Dr. Sebi taught, I began looking into alkaline foods.

The next order of business was to study the foods that were harmful to my body. Brione, as well as one of my best friends had been urging me to view a documentary called "What The Health". I was once afraid of watching it due to what I may hear but I was desperate and I needed to equip myself with as much knowledge as possible to fight this illness. "What The Health" was very informative. I understand that it is an edited motion picture so not everything in it can be 100% true. However, everything had at least some truths, and it opened my eyes. I learned about how animal protein was the main culprit for a vast majority of the sicknesses and illnesses we face in our world today. Animal protein was aiding in the creation of excess mucus in my body. I was grateful to be aware of what was out there. I continued doing my own research and concluded that I would have to make a drastic change on my diet. Much more of a change than I originally thought.

In my thinking, I couldn't just take the information I learned in one documentary, I had to find another. I needed to see if others not only thought similarly but were courageous enough to shed light on that thinking with a documentary as well. I discovered a documentary called "Forks Over Knives," and watched it immediately. It was quite informative. I saw studies done at top medical centers in the country. I saw non-traditional doctors helping others to not only heal but also reduce or eliminate their use of prescription medication all by changing what they ate. I saw testimonies of people having lost weight, gained a great level of normalcy in their blood work, began sleeping better, functioned through the day, and reduced or eliminated pain and symptoms. It was a beautiful thing to witness. One of the doctors shared the results of a study he'd conducted with mice. He gave a group of rats, Group A, a primarily plant-based diet with only 5% animal protein. He gave Group B 20% animal protein in their diet. All the rats were of good health at the start. As the weeks passed, the doctor noticed that Group B, with 20% animal protein in their diet began to grow cancer cell. Meanwhile, Group A showed no cancer cell growth at all. The doctor then switched the diets. Group B dropped to only 5% animal protein while Group A increased to 20%. The doctor observed that the cancer cells among the rats in Group B were shrinking while Group A began to grow cancer cells. This led that doctor to conclude that we can turn on and turn off diseases in our body by what we eat. THAT WAS PARAMOUNT FOR ME. By the grace of God I was reassured that I was in control of my progress and that if I was to beat diabetes, I had to make daily decisions.

While I was now getting closer to beginning my virtual workouts and had an idea of how I would eat, I remembered something a doctor had recently shared with me. "If you can lose about 30 pounds, you will give yourself the best chance of managing your diabetes." Now let me be clear, I was not looking to manage ANYTHING! Managing meant accepting that I would have to live with this inside of me for the rest of my life. It meant that excess mucus could never be gone. It meant to me that the symptoms that I had experienced could resurface whenever they felt like it and I would have to learn to deal with them as they come. Managing diabetes was not an option, my goal was to rid my body of it and it not be a concern for me or my doctor. With that said, I realized I needed to give myself a weight loss boost. Here,

I began researching intermittent fasting!

Intermittent fasting, for me, was understanding that I would be restricting myself to when I would eat in effort to maximize the fat that I burned. I saw several options. 12:12, eating in a 12-hour window and for the other 12 hours fasting and only drinking water. 16:8, eating in an 8-hour window while fasting and consuming water only for 16 hours. Lastly, I saw the perfect option for me: 20:4, eating in a 4-hour window and fasting with water only for the other 20 hours. I was **DESPERATE.** So, I went with what appeared to be the hardest option.

The Detox

In the past I subjected myself to the spicy lemonade detox. But I could not put myself through drinking cayenne pepper at a time like this. Therefore, I researched and found a detox that I could be comfortable with.

Initially I took pills that I found online: vitamin D3, turmeric pills, sea moss pills, cayenne pepper pills, and a laxative pill to push out the junk. Now, this was helpful, but it wasn't the most beneficial.

As I continued my research on Dr. Sebi, I found a product on his website called *"green foods"* that I purchased. I began to learn more about sea moss and eventually purchased a jar from some random website that I would not buy from again. I then found what I was looking for, a detox with natural herbs that allowed me to still eat. CRAZY, RIGHT? I always thought there could be no food eaten while on a detox or the detox would not work. I was wrong! The combination of the following herbs went into a smoothie every morning for 10 days straight: prodigiosa, cascara sagrada, rhubard root, duck flower, burdock root, dandelion root, yellow dock, chaparral, eucalyptus, mullein, elderberry, guaco. The smoothie consisted of spinach, mint leaves, frozen pineapples, strawberries, and peaches. I used water from a pitcher with an "alkaline" filter on it (more on that later). Let me be clear, this detox was nasty, even with the fruit in it. However, it was worth it, WORTH IT!

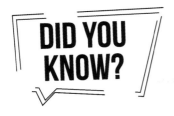

Some High Risk indicators for Type 2 Diabetes:

- Overweight
- Immediate family member with Type 2
- Not physically active at least 3 times a week

Source:

https://www.cdc.gov/chronicdisease/resources/publications/factsheets/diabetes-prediabetes.htm

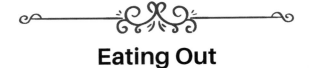

Eating Out

I primarily ate from my refrigerator. I had a tough time starting out. It was challenging to resist my wife's snacks while she was gone, to refrain from ordering from the apps on my phone, or to ignore the temptation of going out to fast-food eateries while my wife was at work. The struggle was really REAL. There were moments of mental breakdowns. I cried with weakness. Not with physical weakness, but with mental weakness. In these moments I wondered if I could really continue to do this regimen, even though it was only for a period of time and not forever. There were nights when I would get up and eat a piece of my wife's leftovers. There were times where I would ask my wife if I could finish her food during the day when she was satisfied. My wife was my rock. Tony Lee and Brione held me down and kept me motivated. My family and friends kept me encouraged. They understood that it was going to take time for me to adjust and get 100% consistent, knowing that I would have weak moments and they were there to lift me up. I am forever grateful to them all.

As the weeks passed, eating out the fridge became more and more normal. I was able to say "no" to my food desires, drinking water to satisfy the majority of moments of hunger. Later in this book I will share with you what I ate and how I ate.

Three month check up

Okay, July 24th I was diagnosed with type 2 diabetes. My A1C was over 15.5, I weighed 275, my blood glucose level was 476 and my Microalbumin/Creat-Alb/Creat Ratio was 168 (which meant I was in early stages of kidney disease). I began intermittent fasting, detoxed my body, ate primarily alkaline foods and worked out 5-7 days a week on my patio. On October 23rd I had an appointment with my primary care physician, Dr. R. I was confident that I had improved, I felt better, I tracked my weight daily and I knew that I had good news awaiting me that morning. Well, while I was waiting to be seen, I randomly checked the mobile app used for all Dr. R patients and I noticed that I had lab result from my April appointment that I had never viewed. As I took a look at them, only one thing stood out and it frustrated me so much. My glucose level on April the 8th was 346. Now for context, the normal range for glucose in the blood is 70-105. I was livid. Although my A1c was not tested on April 8th, my glucose being that high was enough for me to draw the conclusion that Dr. R at least had an inclination that I could have been diabetic. Three months later, July, my blood glucose was tested and 130 points higher. It's a miracle I didn't lose my vision, any function of my limbs or my life. To God be the glory.

Now I'm upset and after my tests for that day showed that I had improved over the last 90 day, I was going to give Dr. R a piece of my mind. Once in his office he informed me that the clinic communicated with him about my diagnosis and he asked me how the medication was going. I responded with, "I don't take medication". We had a brief stare off and then he expressed his disappointment, whatever! I told him I opted to take the natural route and I feel better. Dr. R expressed how the medication was the best thing for my pancreas and kidneys and I needed to take this disease seriously. I didn't respond. I just asked him to test my A1C. I was confident that it had decreased.

A nurse came into the waiting room to speak with me and was rather sad, I assumed she was having a bad day. "Mr. Davis I'm sorry to share with you that your A1C test shows 7.4, but don't worry you can get it down." I smiled so hard!!!! "Ma'am, that is down, you don't understand, I tested over 15.5 three months ago." Her mood changed immediately. She went and told her coworkers. They all came to congratulate me as though I had won an intense game of bingo. Dr. R came back smiling. He stated he saw no need for me to even touch the medication. He recommended that I continued doing exactly what I was doing because it was working!

I also weighed in at 258 on that day and my Microalbumin/Creat-Alb/Creat Ratio was 52. Everything was coming down and getting to normal.

At this point in my journey, I was sleeping better through the night. I didn't need naps. I was hydrated throughout the day and didn't have that "I can't hold it" feeling when it came to my urine. The tingling in my limbs had gone away and I didn't have blurred vision anymore.

Data: Weight, 258lbs. Glucose reading, N/A. A1C, 7.4

Questions:

1. Do you know your current number: A1c, Glucose, Microalbumin/Creat-Alb/Creat Ratio?

2. What plan do you have in place to improve or maintain them?

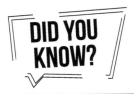

Risk of stroke and heart attack are increased if you have diabetes.

Source:
https://www.cdc.gov/chronicdisease/resources/publications/factsheets/diabetes-prediabetes.htm

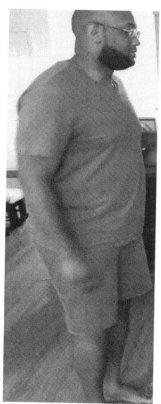

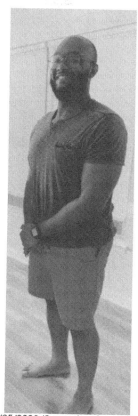

07/13/2020 (2 weeks before diagnosis)   10/25/2020 (3 months after diagnosis)

Tuesday/Thursday:
5:30am wake up and drink water
6:00am-6:20am light cardio in my neighborhood
Shower, hydrate, relax/nap
10am Breakfast: Sliced Granny Smith Apple, 1 cut walnuts, Smoothie
Noon Snack: Low calorie popcorn
2pm Lunch: Salad with grilled chicken (optional)

Not all water is the same

Working from home afforded me many opportunities. I could order things online that I needed for the house. I could clean up on my breaks. I could prepare my meals and monitor what I ate and the times I ate. I also had random ideas. One idea had to do with my urine, "what was the pH level of my urine?" When I checked it I was fairly surprised, it was right at a 6. My goal was to get it as close to 7 as possible. I purchased some pH strips from a popular ecommerce website and had a ton left over. Randomly I thought to test the pH level of the sink water. It was right under 5, acidic. I purchased a water pitcher and decided to test the water that came from it using the factory filter. Now the filtered water I had assumed would have a decent pH level, yet it was also right under 5, acidic. I was a bit stunned, but I didn't let it bother me too much since we drank water from a pitcher and purchased a 3rd party alkaline filter, assuming that once I tested it I would see a pH level at least in the 7s, if not higher. However, I was quite disappointed. The "alkaline" filter produced water that test at a 4.5 pH level, which was......ACIDIC. If I don't recall any exact number, I recall that one. I threw that filter and pitcher out immediately. I viewed it as a hindrance to long term progress since illnesses cannot survive in an alkaline environment but can thrive in an acidic environment. Now I must say, I tested all waters listed above, multiple times. After which I was back to researching water, searching for some that was beneficial and cost effective. I looked into alkaline water, but it was quite expensive for me considering the amount I intended to consume per day, as well as my pregnant wife. No way was I going to allow her to continue to consume something that I determined was not good for either of us. I later met a guy named Paul through a very popular social media site. Paul was very friendly and well versed on the body and what's beneficial vs. what's not. He suggested I consider a certain spring water. I was able to find that water as well as a store brand from a local market. I must say, after testing both, I was well pleased that they were both over 6.5 on the pH scale which was good enough for me.

Since being diagnosed with type 2 diabetes in July 2020, I have only drank water outside of homemade fruit and vegetable smoothies. I push to drink 1.5 gallons a day. I take a half-gallon container everywhere I go, except the airport. I purchase bottled alkaline water if I'm soaring the skies. Since October 2020 I've been consuming a certain spring water only. I trust in it so much; I only bathe my son in spring water.

ALL DRINKING WATER IS NOT THE SAME.

Questions:

1. How do you feel about what you just read concerning water?

2. Do you know the pH level of the water you most recently consumed?

Anthocyanin and spinach

The gentleman Paul I mentioned in last chapter gave me more than just information on water. Paul made mention of colors, colors that would further reshape what and how I ate.

Paul expressed that fruits and veggies that had dark/rich purple, red or blue color was the best for my body. These fruits and veggies are rich in anthocyanin, which is an antioxidant that fights free radicals in the body, and are believed to possess anti-inflammatory, anti-viral and anti-cancer benefits.

When I researched anthocyanin I discovered that it had been used for years to treat blood vessel issue, high blood pressure, and diabetic retinopathy (loss of vision due to diabetes). In addition to that, there were suggestions that anthocyanin was helpful in fighting heart disease.

This information was a game changer for me. Here I am within 14 weeks of learning I had type 2 diabetes and God blessed me with new knowledge that could only help me to get better and better. From that day, my smoothies consisted of blueberries, dark cherries and strawberries. After making that change, I decided to incorporate pure blueberry juice, pure concord juice and pure dark cherry juice and add them to my smoothies as well, in lieu of my spring water.

Shortly after making this change, I discovered a video by Dr. Sebi stating that he does not recommend spinach anymore. He said that in his research he concluded that once metabolized, spinach becomes acidic. I didn't ask any questions, just searched for a green leaf to replace spinach in my smoothies. HELLO KALE!

Questions:

1. Are you aware of the best foods to consume for the health issue(s) that you have?

Turkey Day

Well 4 months in with great progress; I decided to let loose and treat myself. I had been working hard, fighting my cravings (majority of the time), working out consistently and making myself proud. My family was proud, my friends were proud, and I was ready to indulge in the traditional foods for the 4th Thursday in the month of November. I'm talking about, baked macaroni and cheese, sweet potatoes soufflé, corn pudding, barbeque beans, deep fried turkey, potato salad, ham, cakes and pies. I was ready to cut up! Well....I was ready the night before.

On Thanksgiving morning I woke up, stepped on the scale and saw 239.8 pounds. Lord knows I hadn't seen that number in about 5 years. I was excited to keep seeing that weight drop. I did my regular morning workout on my patio. I showered then put on an outfit I hadn't comfortably worn in years. Prior to heading out I thought about the day ahead. I reflected on how I had been feeling over the last few months: light, energized, calm, alert...I wasn't sure I was ready to sacrifice that on today. I didn't think that I wanted to feed my face and deal with instant fatigue and sluggishness, not to mention the great potential of an upset stomach. Before we left home I had a smoothie, which was after my workout. I refilled my water jug and packed me an apple and some walnuts. Once we arrived at our family's home and everyone began to make their plates, I calmly cut my apple and crushed my walnuts into a bowl and sat down to eat. Lord knows I was proud of myself, fighting to have self-control and reassuring myself that food didn't have a control over me, anymore. As the day progressed and we all began to play board/card games, almost everybody began to slowly pipe down; the "itis" was kicking in. I, however, was grateful that I had held out on one of my FAVORITE meals of the year. It was a huge mental milestone for me.

Questions:

1. What is your mentality towards food?

2. What meals, in general, can you delay in effort to heal your body and mind?

3. Have you ever felt that if you skip a certain meal, that you will never have the chance to consume it again?

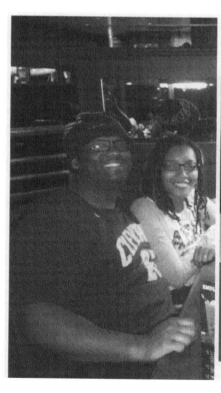
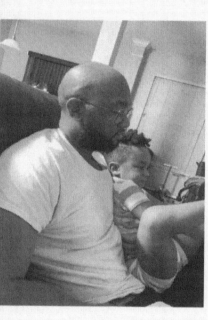

2017 vs 01/2021 (5.5 months after diagnosis)

Monday/Wednesday:

5:30am wake up and drink water

6:00am-6:30am workout on patio with Mr. Lee (jumprope, jog in place, pushups, situps, air squats)

7:00am-7:20am light cardio in my neighborhood

Shower, hydrate, relax/nap

10am Breakfast: Sliced Granny Smith Apple, 1 cut walnuts, Smoothie

Noon Snack: Blue Corn Chips and guacamole

2pm Lunch: Bowl of sautéed veggies with wild rice and guacamole. Grilled Shrimp (Optional).

Apple for dessert

6 month check up

I was approaching my 31st birthday and was excited to meet my new doctor and see what progress I had made. I was excited to finally treat myself to a piece of cake. I can't lie, I did have a piece of lemon cake from Fat Mack BBQ Shack in the Desoto, TX area on my home visit two days after Christmas. I wasn't disappointed in myself, I treated myself to close out the year with a tasty meal with my parents and siblings. I worked out consistently while visiting; training with Mr. Tony Lee was convenient in that way. I also splurged and purchased some bottled alkaline water from a local wholesale store. I had to quarantine from my wife once I arrived back in Virginia and I was disciplined, eating the way I had committed to even with being home alone.

Approaching my birthday gathering, I knew that if I had great documented progress that I could enjoy a piece of red velvet cake from a national Bundt cake maker. I had since left Dr. R for reasons of feeling neglected. I decided to go back to the clinic that originally diagnosed me since my insurance allowed for me to utilize them as my primary care physician. I approached my appointment with my new doctor with confidence and it was SHOT immediately. After the nurse came in to take my blood and urine sample, the doctor came in. She asked me "Mr. Davis, how's it going taking the diabetes medication?" With a sense of pride, I replied "Oh no, I never took that stuff." There was an awkward silence that was so loud enough to mute my bright yellow shirt. She didn't say anything, not a word. The doctor turned around and walked out the room for about 15 minutes. All I could think to myself was, "I'm making a bad first impression." After initially feeling a bit insecure, I regained my composure and took a grasp of the confidence in my approach to fighting this illness and taking responsibility of my own health.

When the doctor came back in, she was beaming. Her smile made me smile as I had assumed she had good news. She began talking about how she saw my records from 6 months ago and was disappointed that I could be so careless to not take the diabetes medication but she didn't want to say anything until she saw my test results that day. She said she was not only impressed but encouraged to see that my blood glucose had decreased from 476 in July 2020 to 118 in January 2021. My urine pH level was now 6.5. My A1C level was GREATER THAN 15.5 in July 2020 and in January 2021 got it down to 6.1. When asked what I did, I told her upfront, "I took responsibility for my own health." I then went into detail of all the changes I made and why. She was in shock. "Mr. Davis, we don't see turn arounds like this, this is very rare. Most patients take the bad news of the diagnosis and either eat the pain away or ignore it and continue with their lifestyle. What you have done is something that is uncommon, you should be the poster child for fighting diabetes. I am very proud of you and hope you keep up the good work." It was later communicated to me that all my organs were beautiful, no fear or concern of kidney disease.

I left the doctor's office, elated! I called my parents and my wife to share with them the great news. I had made a friend through social media, OC, and shared my results with him. My friends and relatives were all called within a matter of days. They were so encouraging and supportive. On my birthday I enjoyed that cake!

I must mention that even at the time of this writing, I have yet to enjoy a tasty bowl of punch. The juice my Mother-In-Love and Sister-In-Law make on holidays and birthdays always looked and taste amazing but I couldn't bring myself to take a sip. I know that of all the items I gave up, soda and juice were the two things that would undo everything for me. I couldn't drink either in moderation so I've only drank water since my diagnosis in July (spring water and occasionally alkaline water since October) and home made fruit and veggie smoothies.

Data: Weight, 237lbs. Glucose reading, 118. A1C, 6.1

Questions:

1. What is your greatest fear when it comes to diabetes for either you or your loved one(s) that may have diabetes?

2. What is your second fear?

3. Do you believe that you can rid your body of this illness and heal from the inside out?

4. If you are not taking diabetes seriously, what are your concerns?

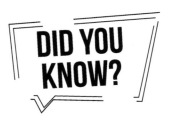

88 Million Americans have prediabetes

- Only 10% are aware

Source:

https://www.cdc.gov/chronicdisease/resources/publications/factsheets/diabetes-prediabetes.htm

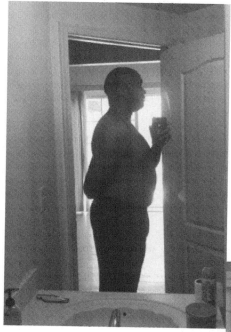

<----08/09/2020
(2 weeks after diagnosis)

01/30/2021 (6 months after diagnosis) ---->
Shirt Size L, Jeans
38 waist

Sample grocery list:

Kale (or any leafy green), Frozen Fruit
(strawberries, blueberries, black cherries,
mango). Fresh Granny Smith Apples.
Spring Water. Burro bananas (fried in
grape seed oil). Spring salad mix. Frozen
shrimp. Chicken breast. Fresh veggies (bell
pepper, onions, squash, zucchini,
cucumbers, tomato, eggplant). Wild rice.
Blue corn chips and guacamole. Low
calorie Popcorn. Veggie nuggets.

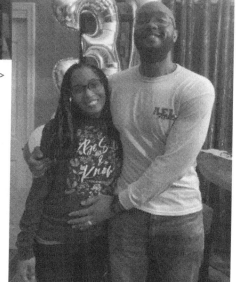

Consistency / Accountability

This journey has been a challenge, each and every day, even now as I am writing this. There were days that I broke down emotionally and cried to God and my wife. There were days that I thought, "I can't do this." There were days where my trainer would introduce an exercise or increase the intensity and I doubted myself. The reason I have had success in healing my body of type 2 diabetes is because of God's grace and the support system He placed around me. My wife, family, friends, trainer and herbalist all held me accountable for my actions in favor of or against my own body. Random text messages asking me what I ate today, or how much water have I consumed were helpful and appreciated even if I didn't want to respond. Talking to my cousin almost every morning aided in my consistency. I knew when we talked every morning he was going to ask me if I had worked out. I was fortunate to have my cousin go on this journey with me from a distance, changing his diet, working out in support of me and being by my side. As difficult as it has been, it's possible with God, consistency and accountability.

Consistency doesn't mean perfection, AT ALL! Every day, every hour, every moment you have a decision to make. Once the decision is made, it's made, you move on to the next decision and so on and so forth. I fell off the wagon at some point every week. If it was taking a bite of my wife's chicken sandwich or finishing off her leftovers late at night. Ignoring my specific snacks in the middle of the day and taking handfuls of my wife snacks. Getting emotional and ordering food through a popular app on my phone. There are a number of decisions that I wish I had made differently but once they were made, they were made and you can't take them back or redo them. Take it one day at a time and stay levelheaded.

Accountability is essential, if nobody knows what you are going through on this journey, chances are you may not do as well as you'd like. Accountability is tough, but it's a key component in healing your body. I'm not saying talk to everyone, what I am saying is lean on the folks in your corner that want to see you achieve what it is that you desire as it relates to combatting this illness. It does require full transparency. It's worth it, I assure you.

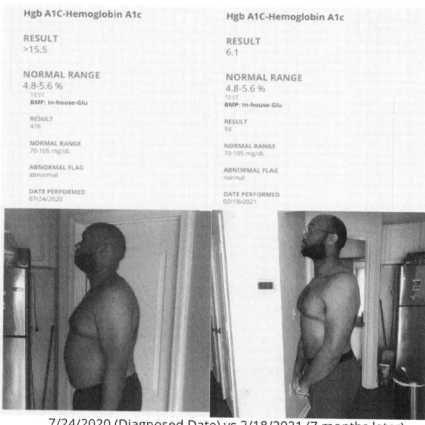

Hgb A1C-Hemoglobin A1c

RESULT
>15.5

NORMAL RANGE
4.8-5.6 %
TEST
BMP: In-house-Glu

RESULT
476

NORMAL RANGE
70-105 mg/dL

ABNORMAL FLAG
abnormal

DATE PERFORMED
07/24/2020

Hgb A1C-Hemoglobin A1c

RESULT
6.1

NORMAL RANGE
4.8-5.6 %
TEST
BMP: In-house-Glu

RESULT
93

NORMAL RANGE
70-105 mg/dL

ABNORMAL FLAG
normal

DATE PERFORMED
02/18/2021

7/24/2020 (Diagnosed Date) vs 2/18/2021 (7 months later)

Saturday:
7:30am wake and drink water
8am-8:30 am light cardio in my neighborhood
shower hydrate relax/nap
11am Breakfast: smoothie
2pm Treat day: small portion of enjoyable meal.

Sunday:
5:30am wake up and drink water
9am breakfast: smoothie
11am Lunch: Salad with grilled chicken (optional)
1pm Late lunch: Banana fries and veggie nuggets
4pm optional snack: Low calorie popcorn or blue corn chips
with guacamole

9 month check up

Continuing on with being consistent, I was still riding the high of my improvement from January, three and a half months later. I continued working out consistently through the week, keeping up with my spring water and sea moss gel plus herbs and still choosing to keep a primarily alkaline diet. Going into my April appointment, now 9 months after my official diagnosis, I was expecting to see similar numbers to January. I went back to the same clinic as I did for my 6-month checkup and was pleased to hear that my numbers remained consistent to that of my last visit. My A1C remained at 6.1, my glucose level dropped from 118 to 87, my kidney function was normal, Microalbumin/Creat-Alb/Creat Ratio was 25 (when I was diagnosed in July of 2020 it was 168), Fasting Lipid Panel-Cholesterol, Total was 105 (it was 70 when diagnosed in July 2020).

The doctor I saw on that day was also impressed and curious as to the changes I made to which I shared. He not only echoed how such improvements in a short amount of time isn't normal, he also expressed his excitement for my not taking the diabetes medication. He said that he has seen an increase in kidney dysfunction for patients on that particular medication.

I walked out of that office with my head held high. I wanted to keep this level of health and so each day I have a choice to make.

Data: Weight, 255lbs. Glucose reading, 87. A1C, 6.1

Questions:

1. When are you going to go all in on improving your health?

2. What, if anything, is holding you back?

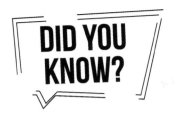

27.2% of African Americans with diabetes have some mild to severe form of visual impairment.

Source:

https://minorityhealth.hhs.gov/omh/browse.aspx?lvl=4&lvlid=18

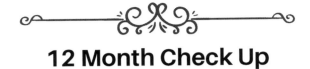

12 Month Check Up

Last chapter was full of joy for me! I had a great visit. My numbers were similar to my 6-month checkup and I felt great. Three days after my 9-month visit my son was born and my world felt complete. It was a great week to have risen above a self-inflicted illness just in time to give love and attention to my son and wife after delivery.

Fast forward 3 months later at my next checkup, I was knocked off my cloud. I discovered that my A1C rose from 6.1 to 7.1 and I felt defeated. I couldn't understand what took place or where I went wrong. A year after my original diagnosis I was supposed to continue making progress, not taking steps back. Needless to say, I shed a tear on my way home wondering how I was going to break the news to my wife.

Once home, it took a few minutes, but I just blurt it all out and afterwards I was reminded why I feel in love with my wife. Soon as I finished, she smiled and simply replied, "we just had our first child." At first, I didn't understand, I could never point a finger of blame towards my family for my health, especially not my baby. My wife broke down the last 3 months for me. With the life-altering blessing we were off all of our normal routine. We had takeout almost every day. We hardly slept the first two weeks he was home so naturally I had no energy to neither workout nor shop for groceries. In the middle of the night when our son would nap longer is when I found time to eat anything I could find in the pantry.

After that conversation I spoke with both my mom and mother-in-love, both of whom shared the same thing with me "you had to experience this for your testimony." Initially it was tough to accept but once I calmed down and took those words to heart. I saw the silver lining. Everything I had done the nine months prior to the birth of my child can now be put to the test. I was back up to 260 pounds and my A1C was 7.1. I decided to get back to my routine and reduce both those numbers by my next appointment in 3 months.

Data: Weight, 260lbs. Glucose reading, 102. A1C, 7.1

15 month appointment

Desperation is a feeling I have gotten used to. In fact, I need it to actually get some things done. In desperation I wanted to try something new that I had frowned upon for years. I began juicing. In my one-on-one session with Godlyherbs.com I learned that the nutrients in the fruits and vegetables that are consumed from juicing are of a higher concentration and get absorbed into the body much quicker since the fiber is removed. I must say I didn't fully understand that but through my research I learned to trust it. Therefore, I added it to my regimen. I would make my juice out of alkaline fruits and vegetables every morning and drink 8-12oz twice a day.

Mr. Lee, my personal trainer, kicked up my workouts to focus more on strength while I maintained cardio on my own. We added pull-ups to every session and increased the repetitions of dips and push-ups. We did these with 10-20lbs of added weight with short breaks in between.

I decided to push past my desires and abstained from bread the majority of these 3 months. I made no sandwiches at home, had one burger while out and two burgers at a family function. We ate pizza twice during these 3 months. It was challenging but the weight began to fall off again. I felt inspired to continue. I maintained my consumption of alkaline fruits and vegetables, guacamole and salsa with blue corn chips and 1.5-2 gallons of spring water daily. The natural herbs and sea moss gel were still a part of my daily routine. I didn't have any shrimp in my salad during this time and had candy 2 or 3 times in response to frustration. I also added 1-2 cans daily of hydrogen infused water that I discovered online.

Going into the doctor's office for my next appointment I felt a since of excitement and anxiety. I stepped on the scale and saw that I weighed 236 pounds! That's a loss of 24 pounds from my previous visit. My blood was drawn and my glucose level was 79! That is the lowest I had ever seen! At this point I am feeling excited and happy with my accomplishments. Time passes and the doctor informs me that my A1C level is 5.9! I can't tell you how hard it was to hold back tears of joy. He also advised that I continue with this lifestyle because it is working. Did I mention I have used NO diabetes medication? Just changed my outlook on food and beverages, got into a workout routine, kept my family and friends updated for accountability and put my trust in God for the results I wanted.

This is not the end of this story; tomorrow is a new day and I have a choice to make: keep doing what I have been doing to get where I am now or slack off and live off yesterday's success?

Data: Weight, 236lbs. Glucose reading, 79. A1C, 5.9

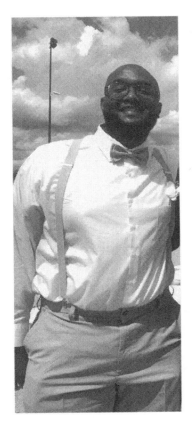

07/12/2020 (2 weeks before diagnosis)
Shirt Size 2-3XL, Pants 44 waist

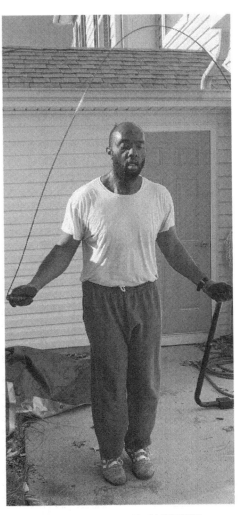

Jumping rope on patio 11/13/2021
(15 months after diagnosis)

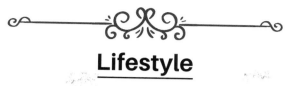

Lifestyle

For about the last 4 years (prior to my diagnosis) I've enjoyed lounging in my free time, playing video games, watching movies and tv shows, eating whatever I wanted and giving minimum effort with trying to work out. I was constantly on the go due to my jobs and so it made it seem as though I was active; however, when I really look at it, I was a couch potato. My free time was truly about relaxing, eating and drinking juices. That was the old me, I don't miss him at all. Since my diagnosis I have been able to enjoy being at home while putting in the necessary work to ensure that I can live comfortably. Working out in the mornings on my patio was embarrassing. I felt weak but little did I know in doing so I was building physical and mental strength and growing in my confidence. I try not to eat late at night still, but I do enjoy tasty things that I like at some point through the week while still maintaining a primarily alkaline diet. I consume sea moss every day multiple times a day and enjoy it. In April 2021, I finally pushed myself to go jog on my own. Having improved in my health and physique actually made jogging enjoyable. I would turn on some upbeat music and push it for 8-12 minutes and then I was done. I don't have the need to work out for hours at a time; I learned that 30 minutes a day was enough to get me the results I desired. I still only drink spring water as I'm still of the thinking that a sip of juice or soda will have me hooked and I would eventually go back to one gallon of those a day. Juicing fruits and vegetables or homemade fruit and veggie smoothies are good enough. My mission is to maintain this bill of health so that I can be around for a long time for my family.

The last 3 months I replaced my smoothies with juiced fruits and vegetables. My second cup would be consumed around 3pm.

My goal was to only eat in a 4-hour window each day. Most days I was successful, some days I was not. There were days that I was weak, mentally and emotionally to which I would indulge in a burger and fries or local pizza or simply eating my wife's leftovers. However, I was consistent, and consistency is what produces long-term results.

One of the more effective strategies that I utilized while eating my meals was watching social media competitive eaters and any videos I could find of them. More often I watched videos of them tackling a timed challenge either in public or in their home. It was oddly satisfying for me and helped me to feel full when I ate the specific meals I ate. Watching videos of these competitive eaters consume insanely large burgers, steaks, pizza, chicken, burritos, nachos, themed dinner plates and even gigantic desserts would trick my mind into not feeling left out but also showing me that I was not missing out on anything.

My final question, are you ready to put in the work to heal your body and defeat this illness?

Please leave us a review on Amazon:
www.tinyurl.com/uncomfortablepeace
or scan here:

Follow and communicate with
Vernon on Facebook and
Instagram:
Vernon P. Davis Jr
@vernonpdavisjr

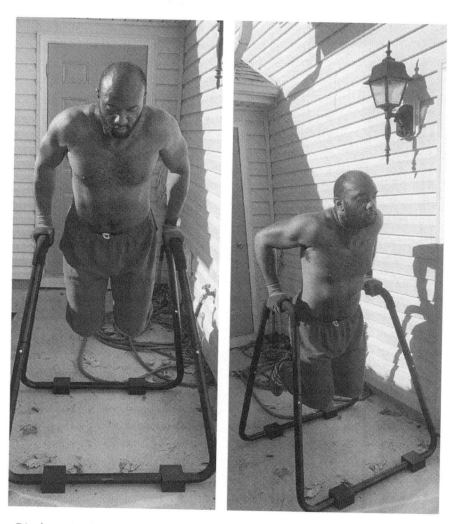

Dip bar workout on patio 11/13/2021 15 months after diagnosis

Made in the USA
Middletown, DE
02 March 2022

61876185R00031